I0711761

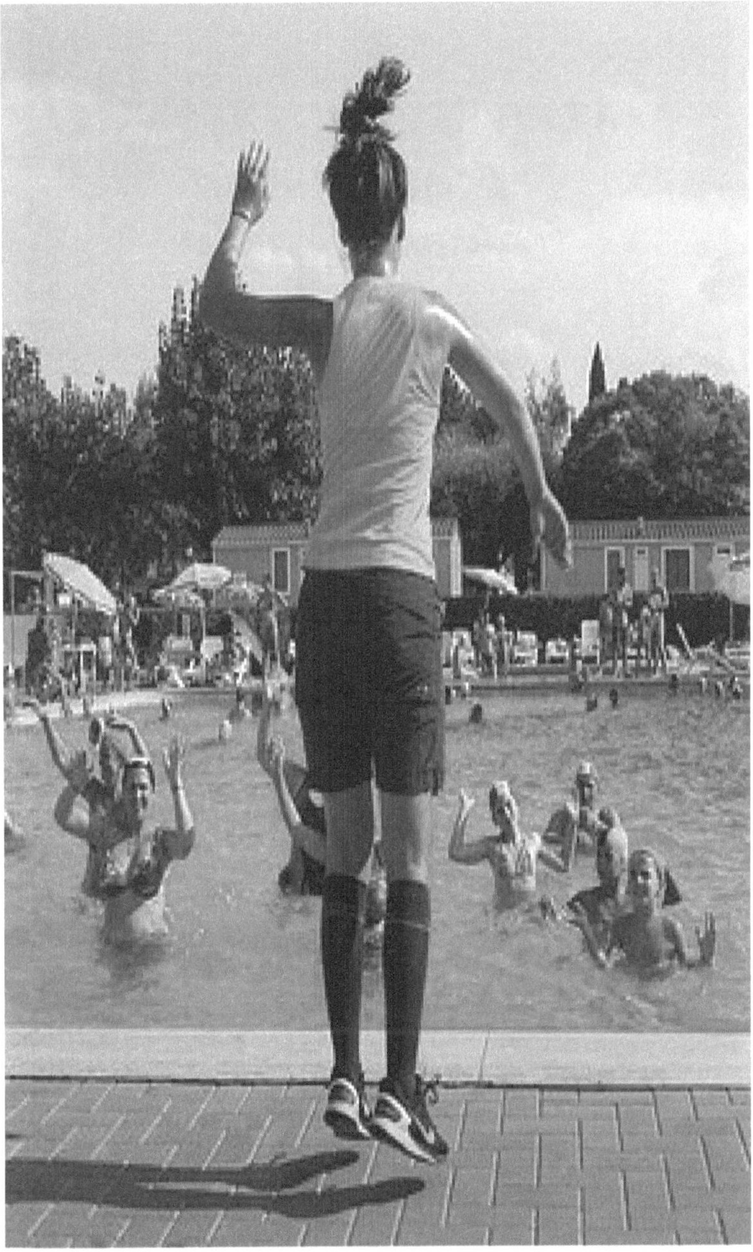

WATER STRENGTHENING EXERCISES

EXERCISES FOR BODY FITNESS, RELAXATIONS, INJURY HEALINGS, AND BODY REHABILITATION.

CHARLES DHARL

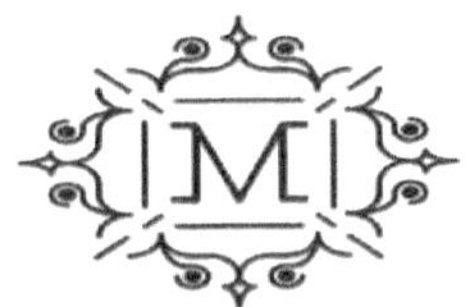

TABLE OF CONTENTS

INTRODUCTION

Besides providing a great place for relaxation, pools are the perfect place to practice some of the best and entertaining workouts since water is up to 1,200 times stiffer than air. Performing your daily routine in a pool is quite beneficial for exercises.

Every time you pull up or push down as well as kick water in the pool you are indirectly performing a lesser pressure of strength exercises and aerobic workouts. This extra work helps you gain more strength, increase metabolism as well as boost your muscles.

In this book we will discuss the various pool exercises for your strength training, boosting of muscles, body fitness, body rehabilitation and injury healings.

Exercise in the pool has another excellent health benefit. Water enhancing simplifies your joints for aquatic training and it also help you to workout with less concern of injury daily by decreasing the impacts of gravity and pressure.

PART 1: BASIC UNDERSTANDING OF POOL EXERCISE

Water exercise is an activity performed in an aquatic environment, such as a swimming pool. Oftentimes, a spa and hot tub can be used for restricted water exercises.

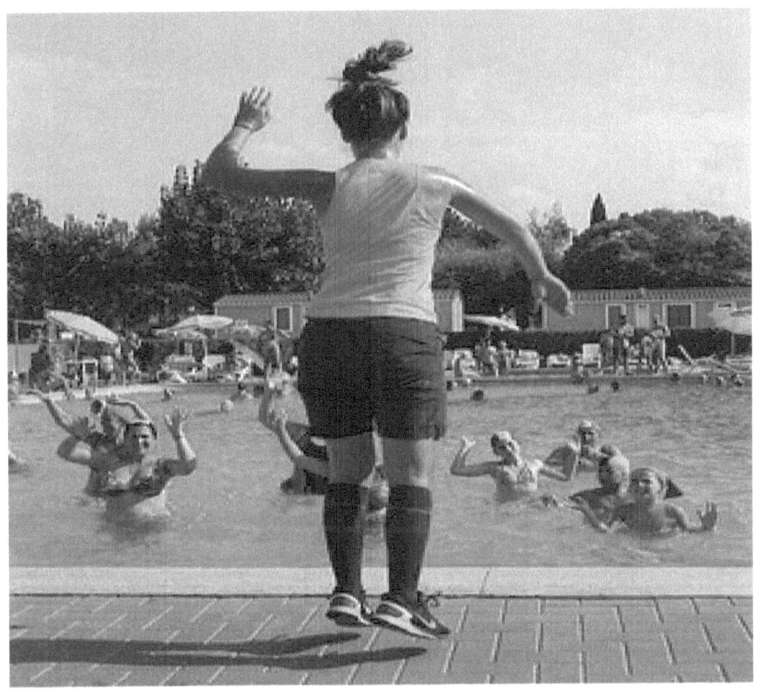

Water exercise is an exercise with a limited intensity that relieves pressure from your bones, joints as well as muscles. Water also provides natural strength that might enhance your muscles.

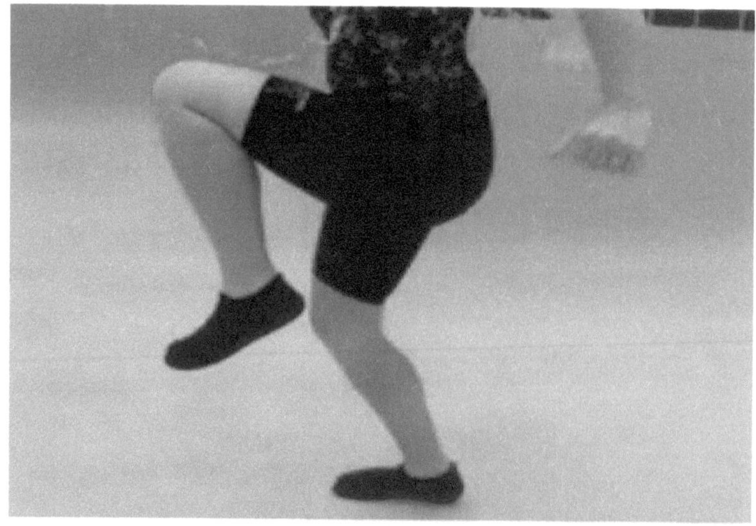

Water exercise can also offer numerous health benefits, including enhancing of cardiac health, less stress, better muscle strength and endurance. Water exercise is one of the best methods to integrate your physical activities. Even if you don't know how to swim you can perform a water exercise but with supervision.

The goal of water exercise is to engage the body into action without placing additional strain as well as pressure on the joints. Although humans have been swimming as well as playing water polo for a great number of years, water exercise evolved out of therapeutic activity for those healing from illness or diseases such as bursitis as well as sciatica.

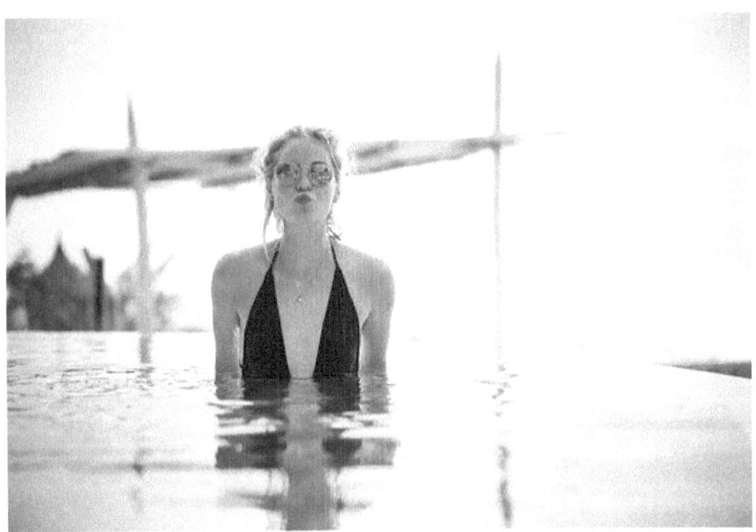

CHALLENGES OF WATER EXERCISE

Older individuals should see their physicians before beginning any fitness program as well as describe the sorts of activities they intend to perform. When beginning a new workout routine, it is essential to begin slowly and gradually increase your intensity. One of the biggest challenges is that, it is not easy to be in control, the flexibility of land exercises cannot be compare to that of water exercises.

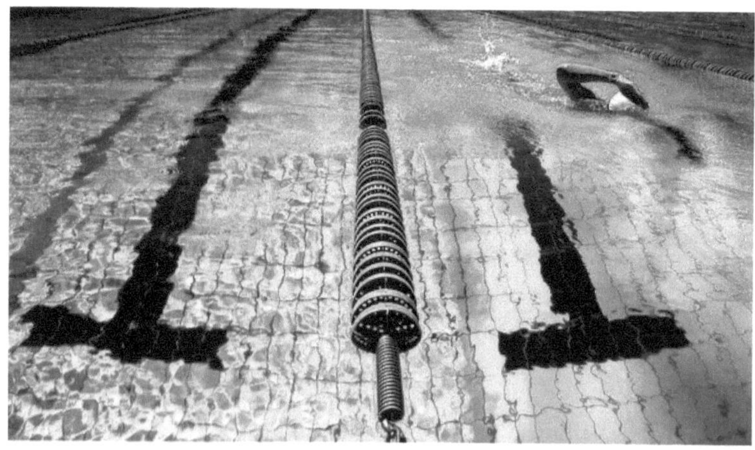

RISKS INVOLVE IN WATER EXERCISE

Since exercising in water is straightforward, novices tempt to overdo it at times that is why it is essential to warm up before beginning. Stretches in the regions that will be exercised should be included in the warm-up routine. Muscle discomfort and aching muscles are two different things that older people should be aware of.

Muscle discomfort is more severe and can persist for up to a week. Seniors should contact their healthcare professionals if this occurs.

PART 2: PHYSICAL PROPERTIES OF WATER

Buoyancies and hydrostatics pressure, as well as viscosities, are three characteristics of water that enable water training safe and secure. These qualities allow us to stay balanced, low-impact workout that is suitable for those who wish to improve their general fitness as well as those who are recovering from surgery or injury.

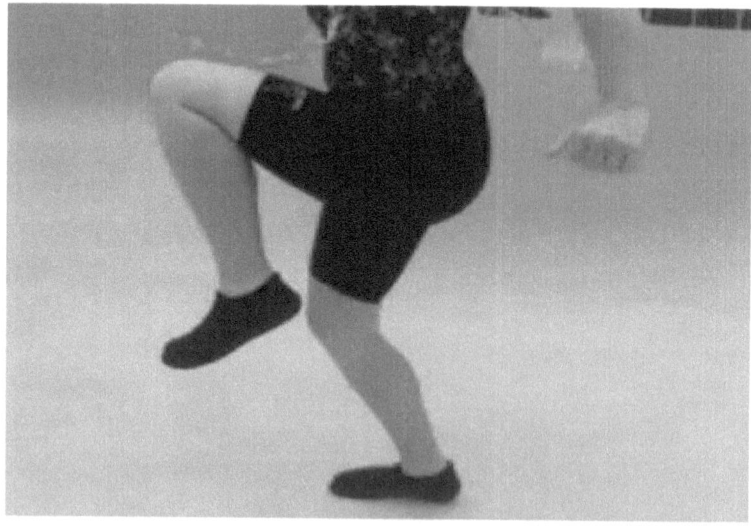

Furthermore, the thermoregulation dynamics in the pool assist to control body temperature, giving water activity a safer and secure atmosphere. Therefore, leading to more enjoyable method of exercise, especially for those with specific health problems like pregnancy as well as fibromyalgia.

VISCOSITY PROPERTY:

Water contains molecules that also offer resistance in both directions, allowing you to simultaneously engage your core muscles.

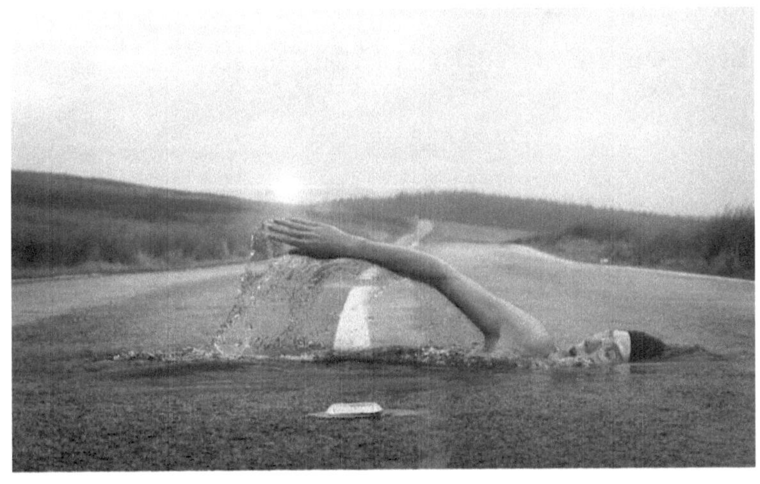

The fact that water molecules are cohesive (that is, they stay together) causes this resistance, which is usually called "drag." To push through some of these sticky molecules, your body needs to expand 15 to 20 times the effort required to move through the air.

BENEFITS OF VISCOSITY

The viscosity of water aids in the building of muscle for your body fitness. It also has a major effect, which allows you to stay upright, making it a safe location to exercise for those who have balance issues, such as numerous different sclerosis and hip replacement.

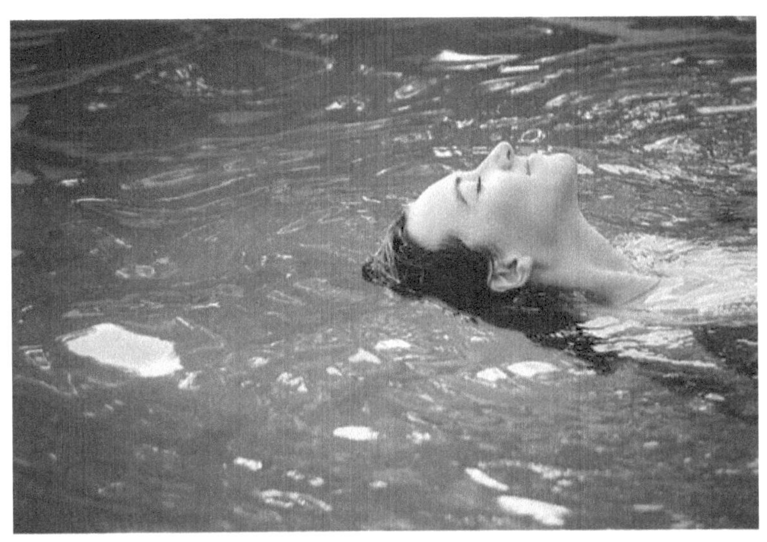

HYDROSTATIC PROPERTY:

The forces applied or transferred by water to an object are known as hydrostatic pressure. The hydrostatic pressure of water molecules exerts the same amount of pressure on all regions of the body, as well as this pressure, rises with deep water.

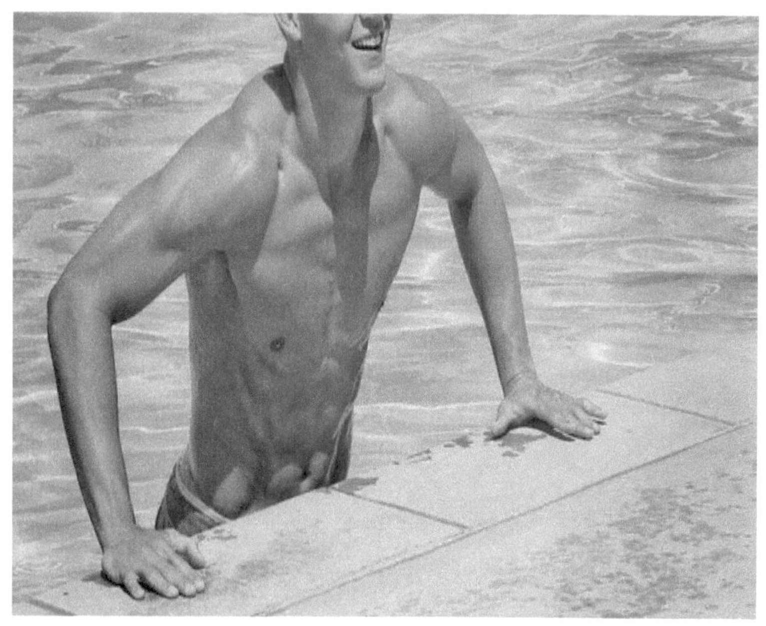

BENEFITS OF HYDROSTATIC

This property of water is extremely beneficial to people who have swelling as a result of an accident, edema during pregnancy, or heart issues. When a joint is submerged in water any edema as well as swelling is reduced because the fluid in the joint is pushed into the capillaries by the hydrostatic pressure of the water on the body, and so returns to the bloodstream. It then travels through the kidneys before being excreted from the body.

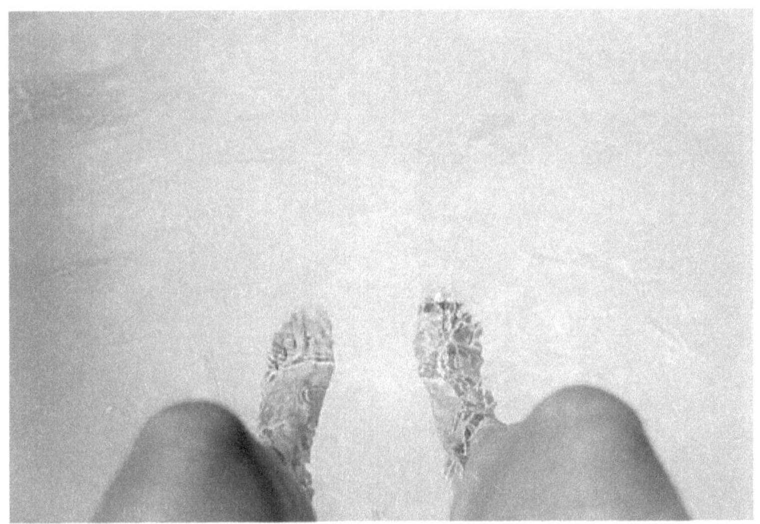

Lower limbs are placed at a higher depth where the pressure is greater. As a result, pregnant women, for instance, experience a reduction in ankle edema.

BUOYANCY:

The most significant benefit of water exercise is buoyancy, which is the upward force produced by fluid—in other words, the polar opposite of gravity's downward pull. Keeping an object, including a playground ball, at the bottom of the pool, then releasing it as well as observing it rises to the top of the water. you can witness the impact of buoyancy.

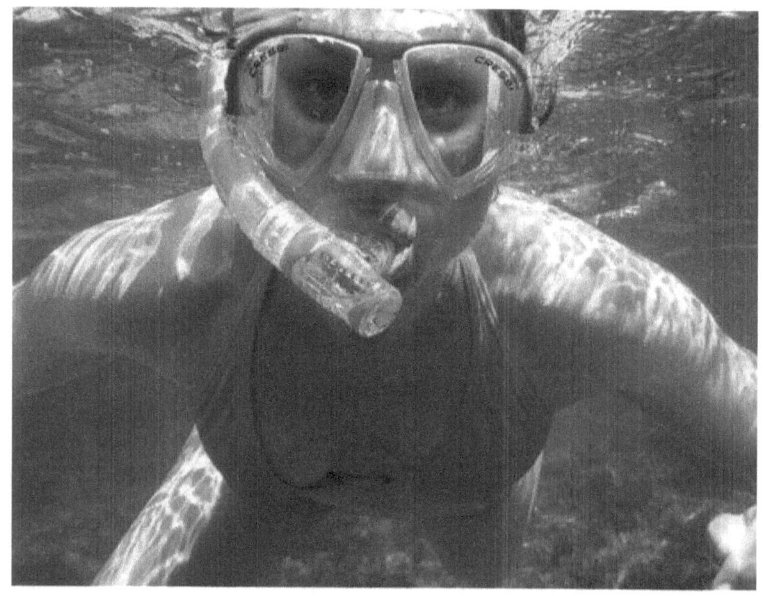

The sense of comparative weightlessness we get while we are in the water is due to buoyancy. It also reduces the compressive pressures that the joints, especially those in the spine are subjected to. Aquatic exercise is thus a low-impact activity.

THERMOREGULATOR:

Thermoregulation is a bodily feature that enhances your degree of comfort while exercising in the pool. The dynamics of thermoregulation in water means that you may control your temperature by transmitting body heat explicitly to the water.

PART 3: BENEFITS OF WATER EXERCISES

The followings are some of the benefits of water exercises:

CHRONIC DISEASES:

Chronic illness patients may benefit from water-based exercise. It enhances the mobility of affected joints in patients with arthritis without increasing symptoms. When people with rheumatoid arthritis participate in hydrotherapy, their health improves more than when they participate in other exercises. Water-based exercise improves the function of affected joints and reduces osteoarthritis discomfort.

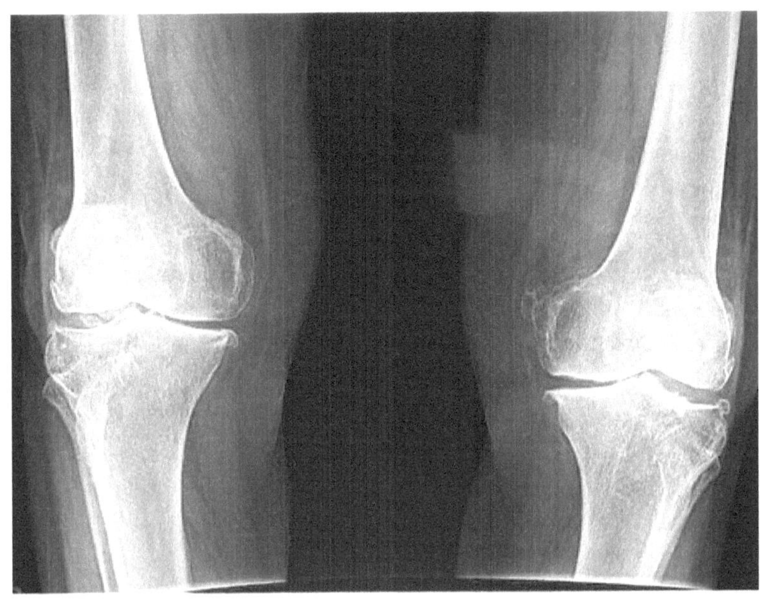

MENTAL HEALTH:

Water exercises are beneficial to one's mental health. Both men, as well as women, can benefit from swimming. It can help patients with fibromyalgia to feel less anxious as well as warm water workout therapy can help with depression. Water-based exercise is beneficial to both mothers as well as their prenatal children's health, also the mothers' mental health. Leisure activities, such as swimming, are beneficial to parents of children with cognitive impairments.

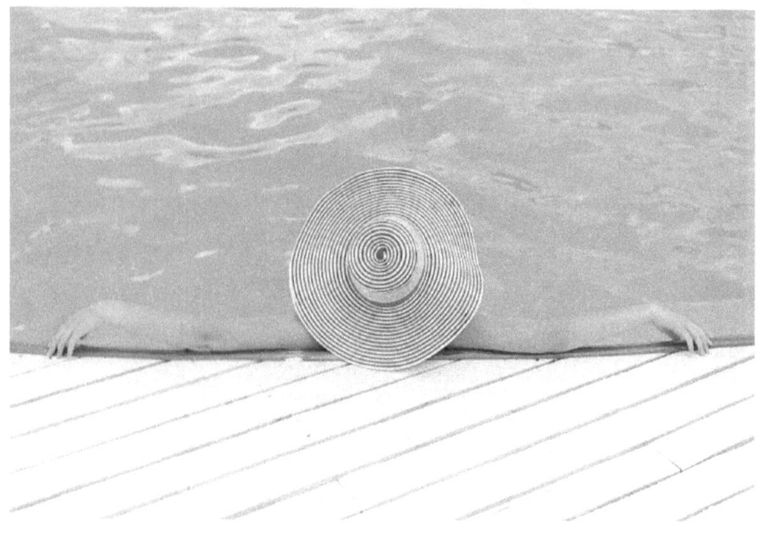

ELDERLY PEOPLE:

Water exercise can help older individuals improve their quality of life while also reducing their injury. It also helps postmenopausal women continuously improve their bone strength.

Exercising in the water has several physical as well as mental health advantages, making it an excellent alternative for those who wish to become more active. When you are in the water, remember to practice safe and healthy swimming habits to keep yourself and some others safe from sickness and damage.

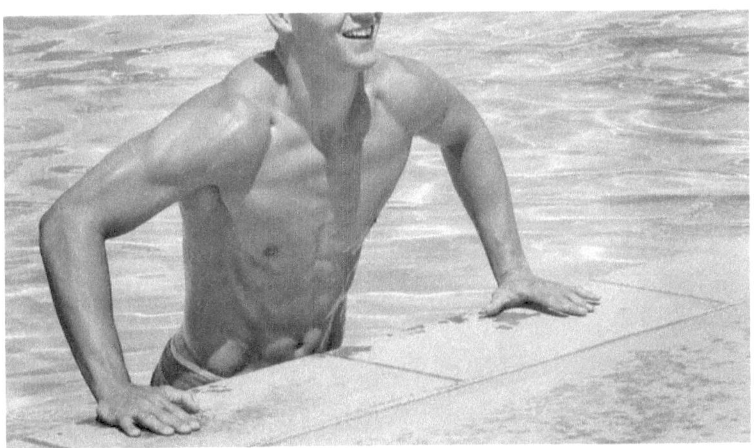

Water fitness programs can assist you to enhance and normalize your heart rate as well as cardiovascular endurance over time. In the pool, the pressure of the water serves as a buddy, assisting in the effective circulation of blood throughout your body.

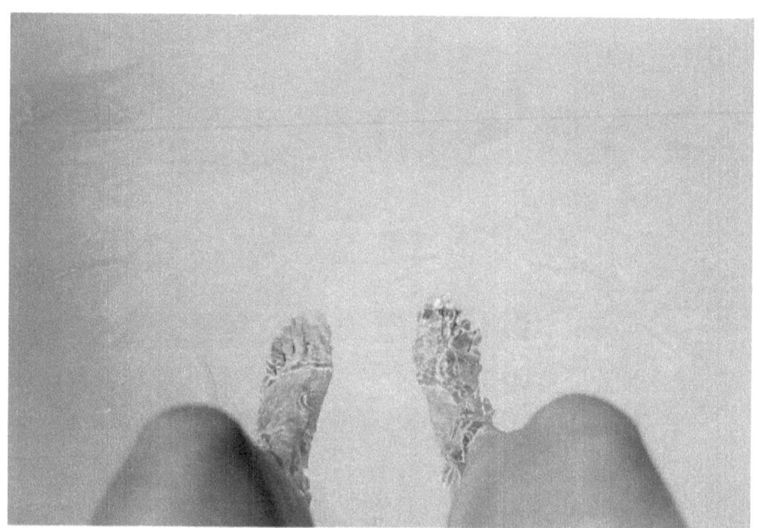

You successfully decrease your risk of heart disease as your heart keeps beating as well as pumping with less strain and pressure. Exercises in the water have even been found to assist those with high blood pressure.

BUILD MUSCLES AND BURN CALORIES:

Water exercise is an excellent method to burn calories as well as tone your muscles. Our bodies, as well as muscles, work more than expected since water is heavier than air and therefore more resistive, resulting in more round and complete exercises.

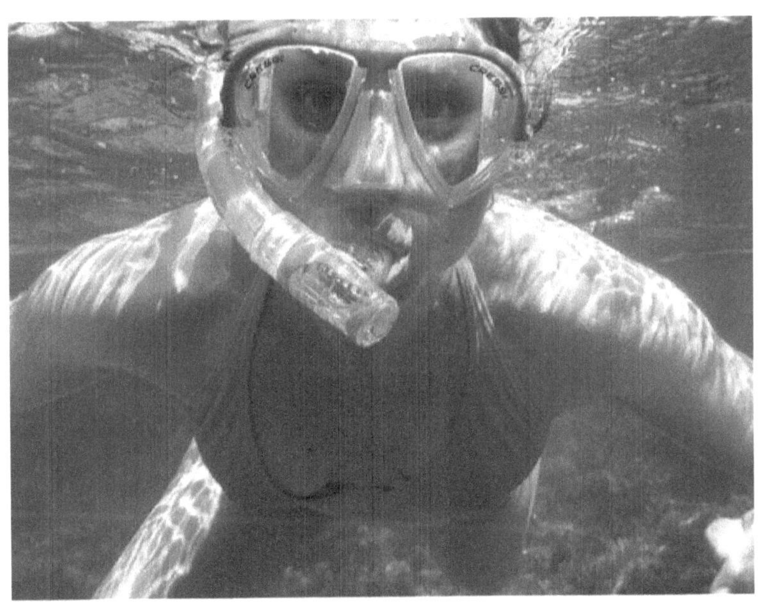

PART 4: GUIDELINES, AND SAFTY

The followings are guidelines for beginners, intermediates, and advanced levels.

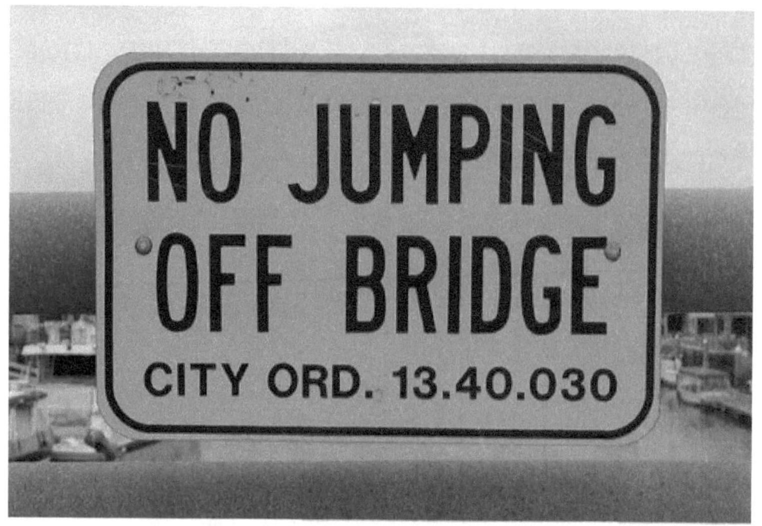

GUIDELINE PROCESS

BEGINNERS LEVEL:

If you are new to the water exercises remember to start slowly. Begin with a 15-minute (or less) exercise; increase the intensity as well as the duration of your workouts as your endurance or strength increases. We also recommend that you exercise 2 to 3 times a week as a beginner and that will enable you to workout at an intensity level of 50% to 60% of your maximum heart rate if possible.

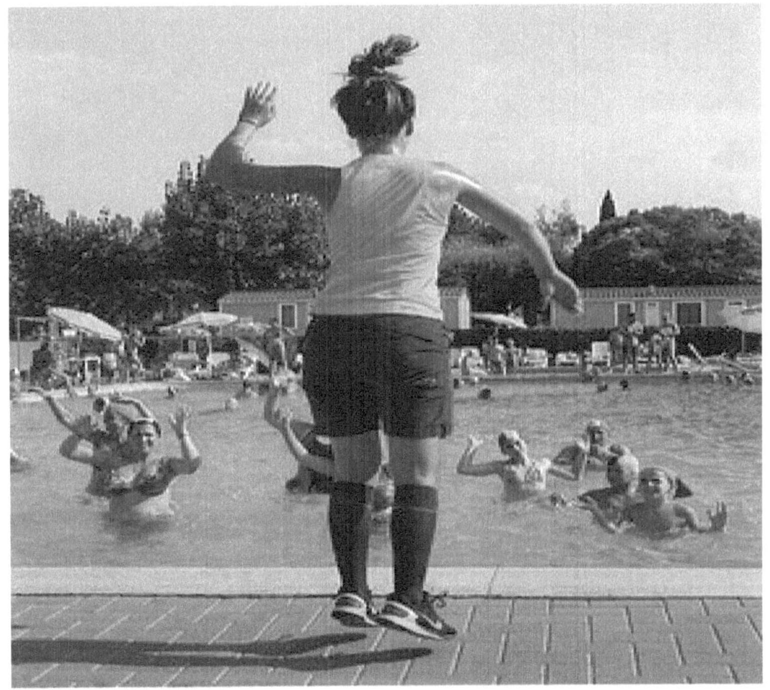

Introduce a few additional exercises as you raise the intensity level of your workouts each week also your endurance level increases. This may be accomplished by increasing the speed and strength of your movements.

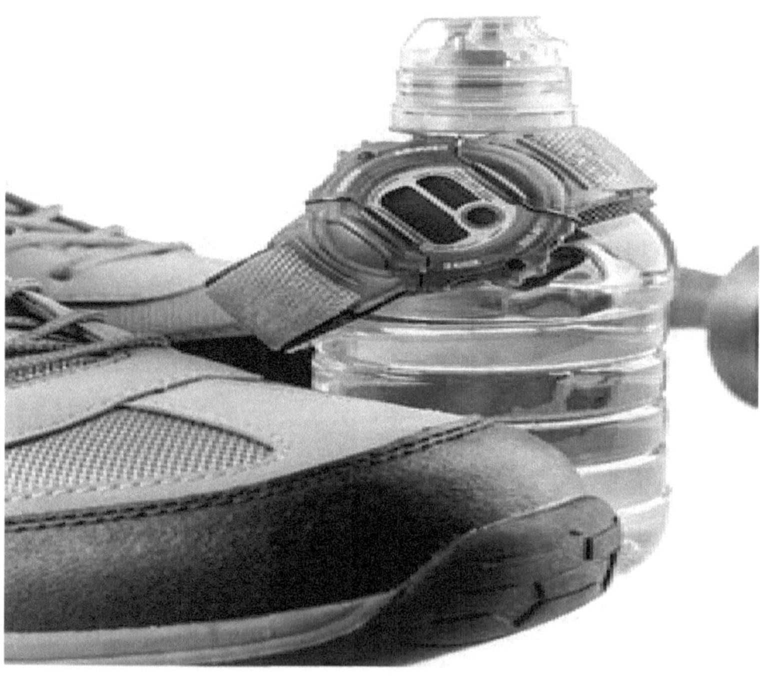

As you progress, you may increase up to 50-70 minute exercises at least four times each week, with the aerobic part of the exercise at 70 to 80 percent of your maximum heart rate.

SAFETY TIPS FOR WATER EXERCISE

Safety is very important aspect you need to consider before you start water exercise. The followings are tips you need to put into considerations:

- Before commencing any workout program, especially water fitness exercises, consult your doctor. If a pre-existing ailment is made worse by your water workout, it might be dangerous.

- Always go through the water training guideline in the water training center.
- Exercise with a partner or at a pool that has an on-duty lifeguard.
- If you are just recovering from injury ensure that you workout with your trainer/coach or you stay in a shallow end of the pool.
- Your water exercise should be tailored to your swimming abilities. If you're not a good swimmer, there seem to be lots of aquatic workouts you may do at the shallow end of the pool.
- Start gently and don't put too much confidence in yourself. It is preferable to move slowly and safely rather than risking an accident in the pool.
- Move out of the water as soon as you feel too hot or cold, disoriented or nauseous, or suffer even a small injury.

- Rather than trying to complete your full fitness routine in one or two days, spread out your water exercises over the week. Trying to exercise for longer period or too hard raises the chance of injury, which can lead to danger of drowning.
- To stay hydrated, drink water before as well as after your water exercise. If you swim in an outdoor pool, avoid doing so during the hottest part of the summer season.

- Study the owner's guidelines for any pool exercise equipment you are utilizing, follow safety recommendations. Only use aquatic fitness equipment according to the instructions in the owner's guidelines.

PART 5: BEFORE AND AFTER WATER EXERCISE.

There are things you need to put into considerations before you start and after you finish your water exercise to maximize the full potential of aquatic workouts.

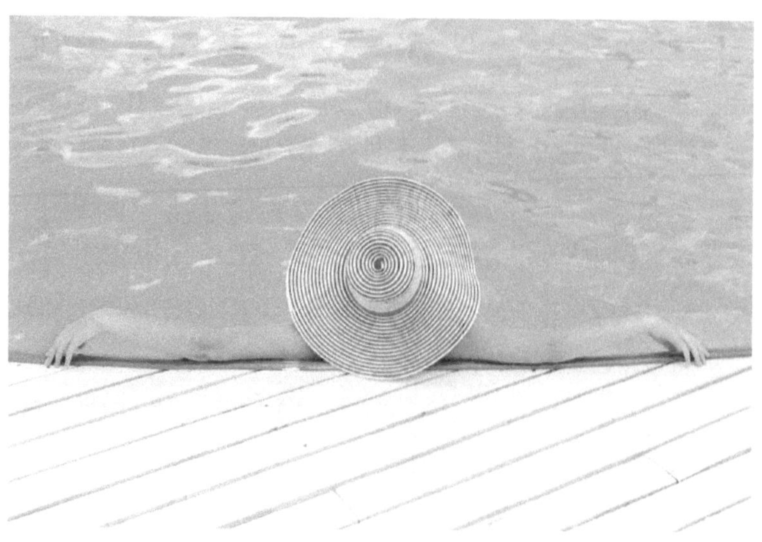

BEFORE YOUR WATER EXERCISE:

GOOD QUALITY SLEEP:

Ensure that you have a good quality sleep this will energize your strength and also make you not to feel dizzy during your exercise.

DRINK ENOUGH WATER:

You probably may be aware that being hydrated is vital for overall health, but it's even more during a workout—since you are sweating both in the pool, you have to make sure your body is adequately hydrated.

LIGHT SNACKS:

Pre-workout snacks can boost your energy for more strength and longevity. You can take some energy drinks and snacks.

WEAR THE RIGHT SWIMMING CLOTHES AND FOOTWEARS:

Being able to jump in the water and move as well as stretch have a lot to do with the kind of wears you are putting on. Wearing a stiff swim truck may limit your flexibility also your footwear has a lot to do with your balance and posture in the water.

PRE-WARM-UP EXERCISE:

Even though your exercise is only 30 minutes long, ignoring your warm-up is not advisable. The warm-up is designed to allow your physique to raise its temperature, boost strength and flexibility, as well as start preparing you for what you are about to accomplish.

AFTER WATER EXERCISE

POST STRETCH EXERCISE:

After water exercise, you can perform post-stretch exercises outside the pool. This will return your body to a resting position.

USE A FOAM ROLLER:

Foam rolling, according to expert as well as some preliminary studies, foam roller can assist you in recuperate from workouts while also increase your range of movement.

It's also recommended by experts as a technique to reduce post-workout pain by boosting blood that flow to the muscles and tissues during exercise. Foam rolling on a regular (and correct) basis can help you heal injuries faster.

POST-WORKOUT NUTRITION:

Pre-workout snacks are more flexible than post-workout snacks. It's necessary to provide your body with the nutrients it requires to recover from hard sweat. Following a strenuous workout, your body seeks carbs and protein to replace glycogen reserves and repair muscle.

LOG AND TRACK YOUR WORKOUT:

Keeping note of what you accomplished during each exercise will allow you to continue to push yourself each time you workout. It's also a wonderful method to ensure that your training program is providing you with the results you desire.

Each week, evaluate what you accomplished and how you felt while doing it to determine whether it's time to go a little heavier, a little quicker, or add a few more reps, or when it's time to slow down and relax and, after a few weeks or months, you will be happy to see all the effort you have put in and the development you have achieved.

CONSIDER WARM SHOWER:

You have been in the water for a long period so you need to consider a warm shower when you get home.

PART 6: BEST WATER EXERCISES

Let's get started with some simple exercises. Now that you have learned about the advantages of water exercise you are ready to get going. The exercises in this chapter are designed to enhance joint range of motion while also causing a slight rise in heart rate. The bulk of these workouts do not necessitate the use of any special equipment. However, once you've mastered the moves, you may use some form of little equipment to enhance the workout's intensity and produce progressive overload.

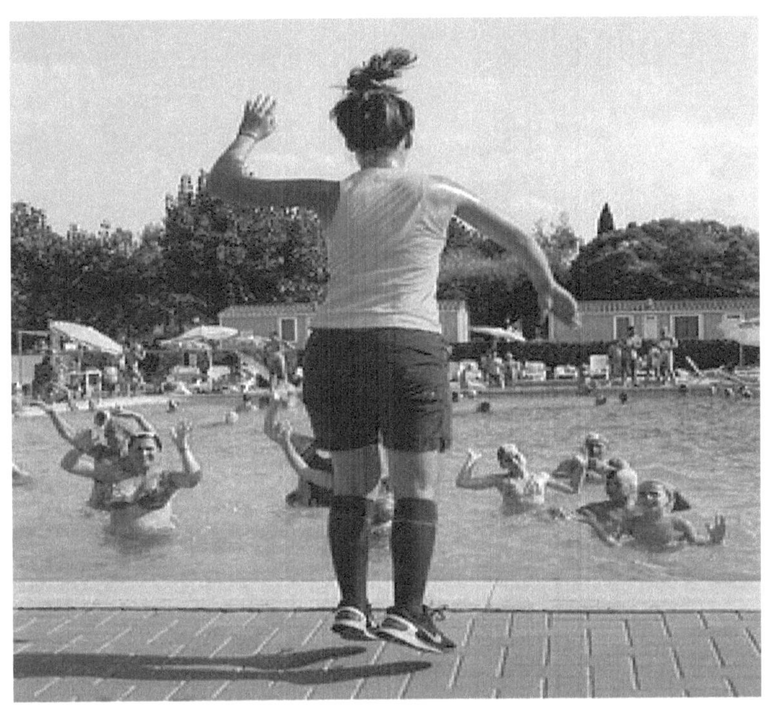

KNEE FLEXION AND EXTENSION

No form of equipment is needed.

This exercise strengthens the hamstrings as well as the quadriceps in the upper leg.

- First, stand straight in the water.
- Your hands should be flat on the side of the wall of the pool.
- Your head and shoulder above the water surface.
- Lift one of your legs at 90 degrees above the floor level.

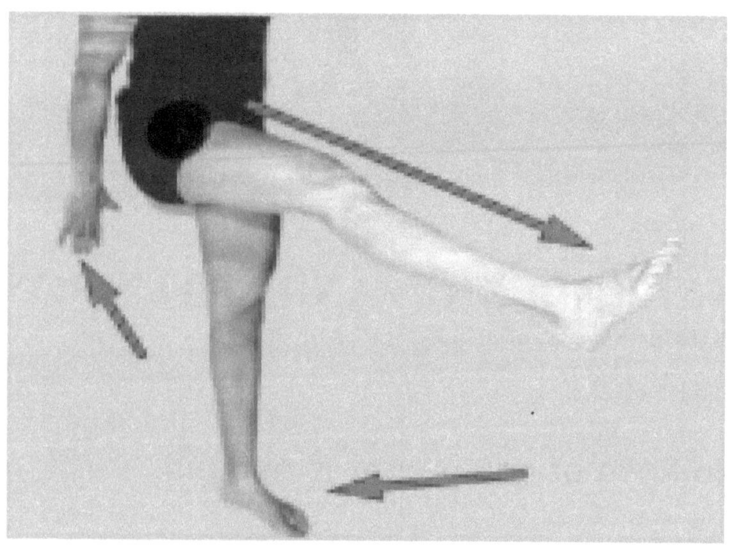

- Now, bent the leg downward from your knee joint but don't allow it to touch the floor.

- After that return your leg straight.
- Repeat the same with the other leg.
- 5-10 repetitions.

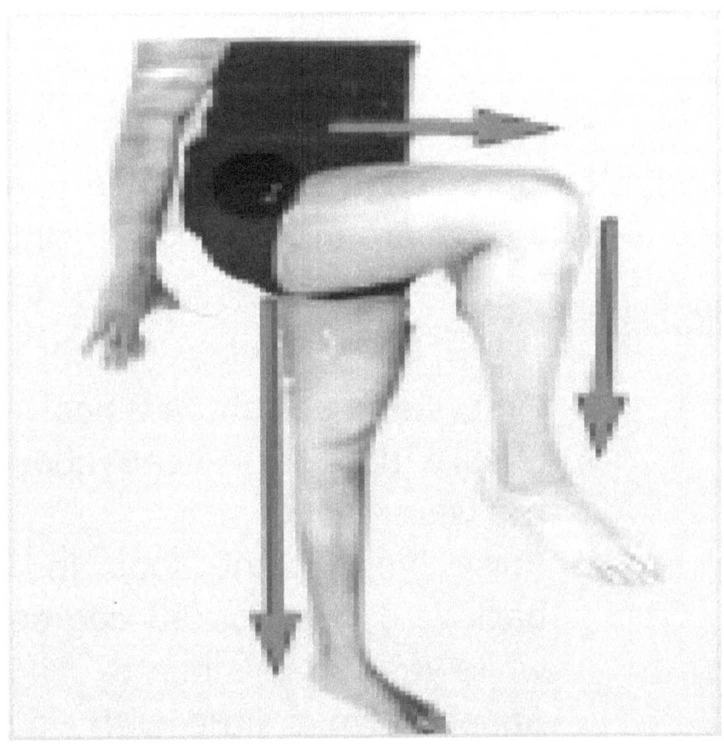

SQUAT SINGLE LEG-UP

EQUIPMENT:

No equipment is needed.

BENEFIT:

Single leg-up strengthen your knee joint and also muscles around your knee joint.

PROCEDURE:

- First, stand upright in a pool.
- Ensure that your head above the water level.
- Raise your right foot in a backward direction 90 degrees while your knee is bent.
- Squat down a little with your left leg and return up while the other leg remains up.
- Repeat the same with the other leg.
- 5-10 repetitions.

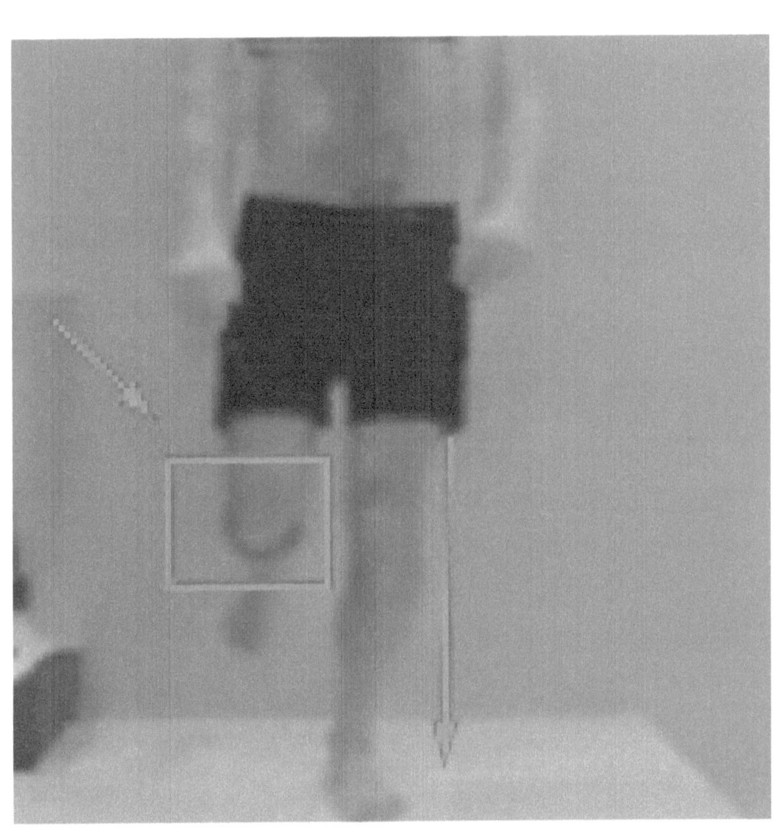

JOGGING SKIP B

EQUIPMENT:

No equipment is needed.

BENEFIT:

Strengthen the muscles of your legs and also your glute. Skip B exercise also strengthens your knee joint because of the pressure and resistance from the water.

PROCEDURE:

- Start by standing upright.
- Hold on the edge of the pool so that you would fall.
- Your foot on the floor of the pool.
- Perform a jogging motion at a fixed place.
- Continue up to 5-10 minutes.

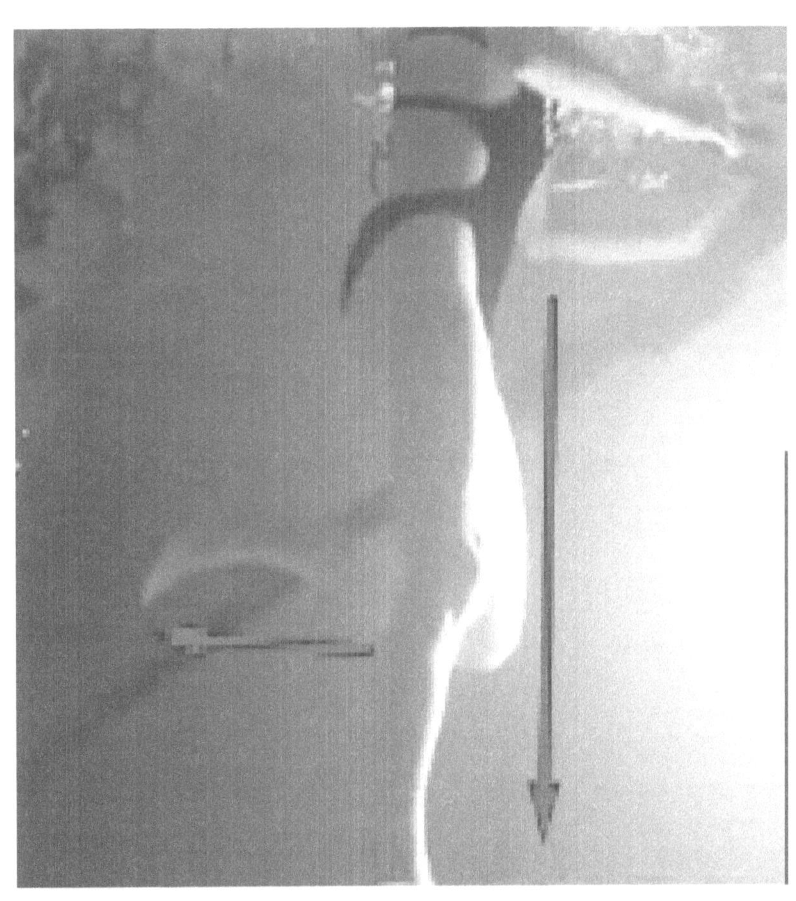

HIP FLEXION

No equipment is needed.

BENEFIT:

This exercise strengthens and also improves the hip flexor as well as gluteus muscles around the hip.

PROCEDURE:

- First of all, stand upright but close to the wall of the pool.
- Your palm on the side of the wall to enable you to stand.
- Your foot on the floor of the pool.
- Thereafter raise your left leg straight and return to the original position.
- Repeat the same with the other leg.
- 10-15 repetitions

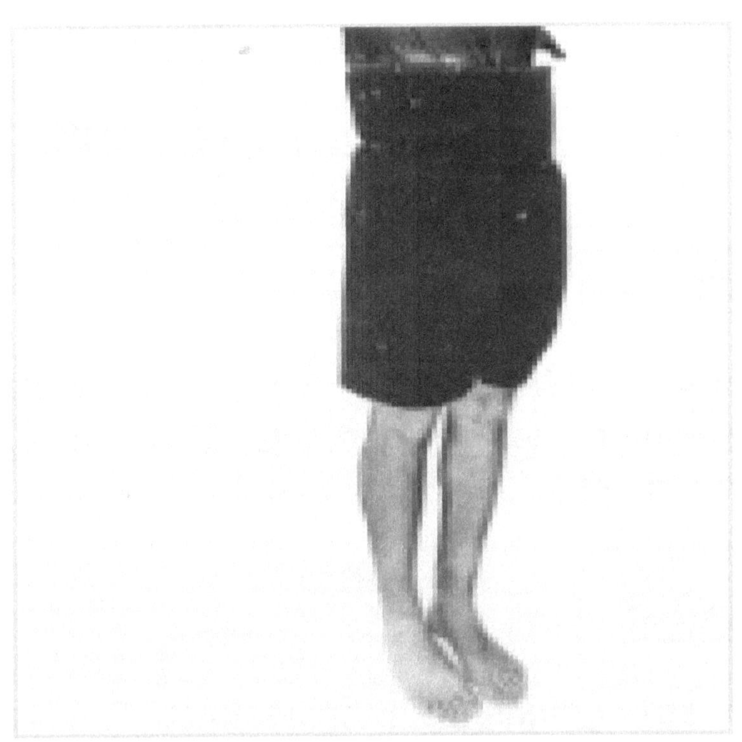

HEEL BACKWARD AND HEEL BEHIND

EQUIPMENT:

ANKLE WEIGHT FOR AQUA (this aqua weight comes in four sets, two are for the hand weight and two for the ankle weight).

BENEFIT:

It strengthens your ankle joint. Due to the pressure on the legs, it also helps to strengthen knees and glute the muscles around the leg region.

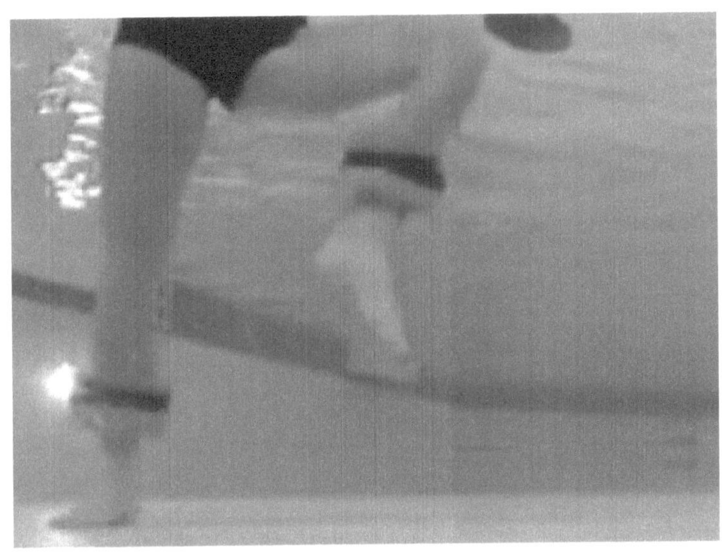

- Firstly stand upright with your feet on the floor of the pool.
- Place the ankle weight on both legs while you hold on the hand weight.
- Be in motion by jogging while jogging in the pool this will put a lot of pressure on both legs then raise your left leg behind to touch your right hand also do the same with your right leg to touch your left leg.
- 10-15 repetitions on both legs.

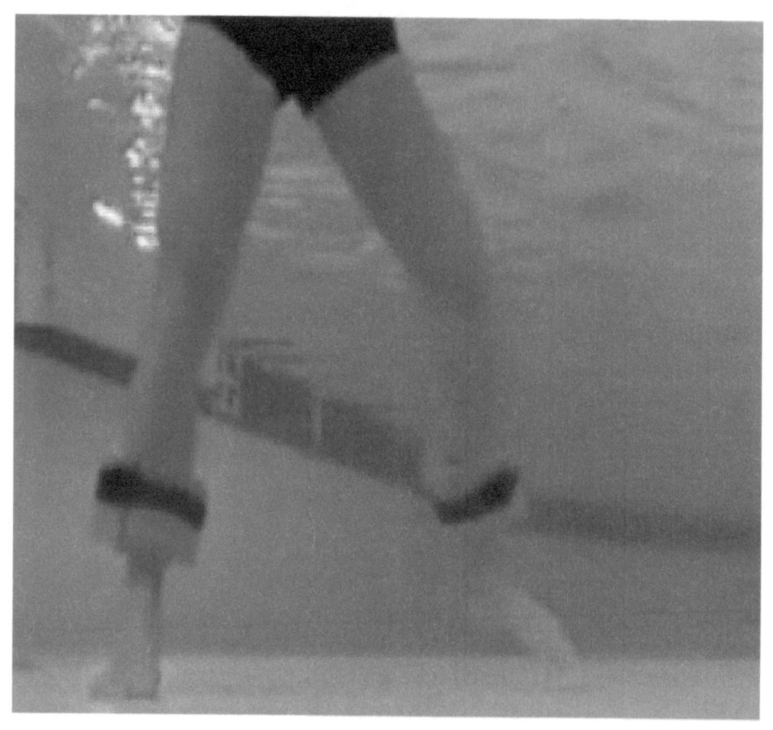

HIP EXTENSION

EQUIPMENT:

No equipment is needed.

BENEFIT:

It helps to activate and strengthen the flexors and gluteus muscles of the hip.

PROCEDURE:

- Start by standing upright.
- Your foot on the floor.
- Your hands-on edge of the pool.
- Your head and shoulder above the water level.
- Lift your right leg backward and return to the original position. Do it again.
- Repeat the same with the other leg.

- 15-20 repetitions.

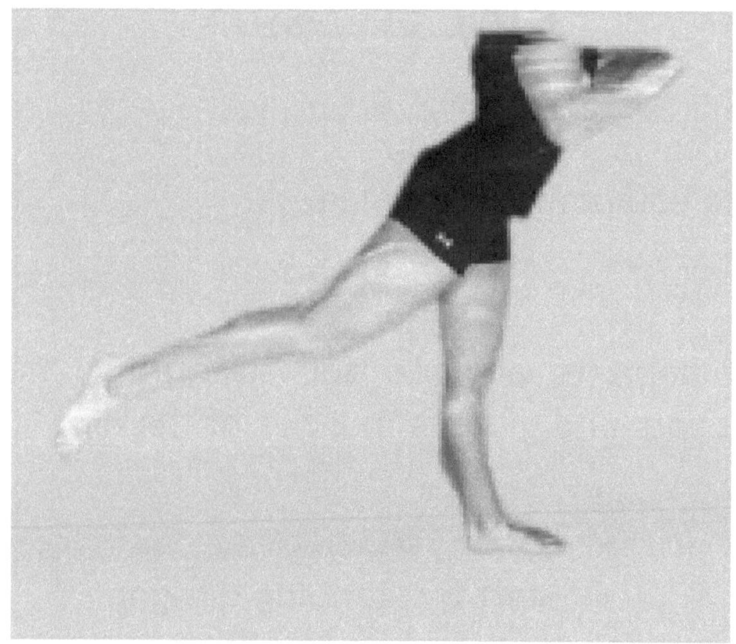

ACQUA JOGGING

EQUIPMENT:

No equipment is needed.

BENEFIT:

It helps to strengthen the bone because water jogging involves a weight-bearing workout that also enhances cardiovascular fitness.

PROCEDURE:

Perform regular jogging exercises but this time in the pool. 10-20 minute jogging. 2 sets

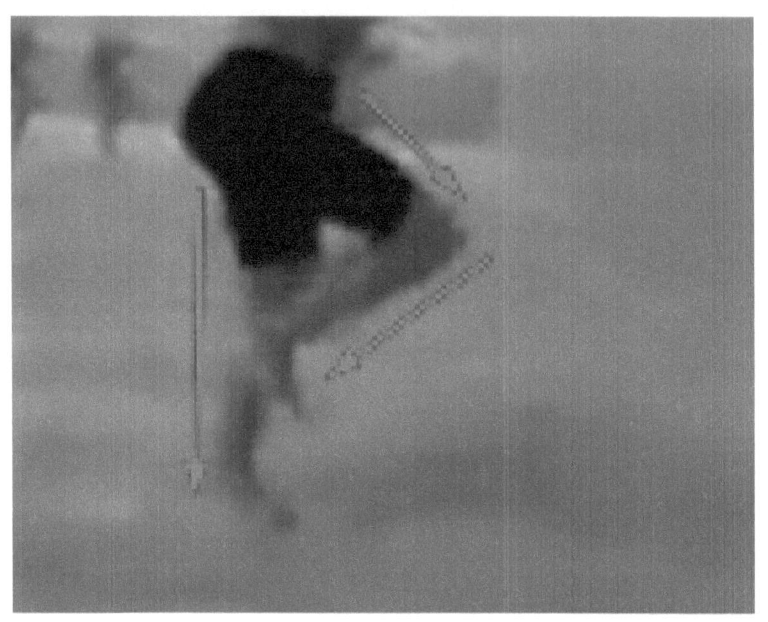

FORWARD AND BACKWARD LEG SWING

EQUIPMENT:

No equipment is needed.

BENEFIT:

This exercise focused more on the muscles at the front and back of your hip as well as your upper leg.

PROCEDURE:

FORWARD SWING:

Firstly stand upright in the pool. Lift your leg from your hip forward at 90 degrees. Swing backward without the leg touching the floor.

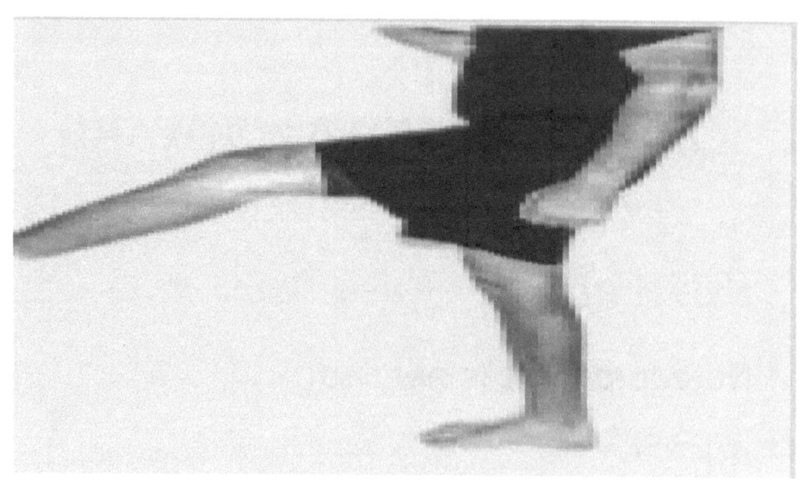

Repeat the same thing with the other leg.
10-15 repetitions.

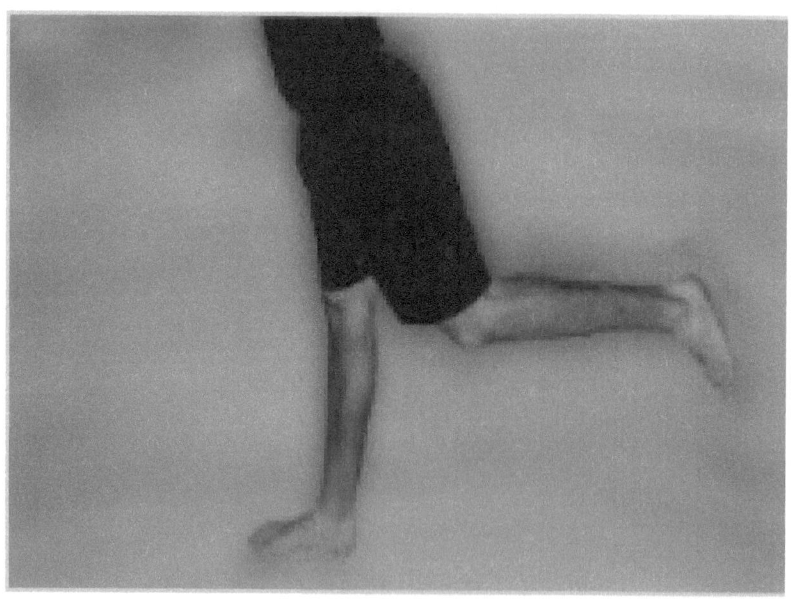

WATER KICK

EQUIPMENT:

No Equipment is needed.

BENEFIT:

It activates and strengthens the muscles around your hip and also gluteus.

PROCEDURE:

This exercise is done by raising one of your legs and performs a leg kick on the water. First your raise your leg up and perform a kick in the water. This exercise is sometimes difficult due to the resistance from the water.

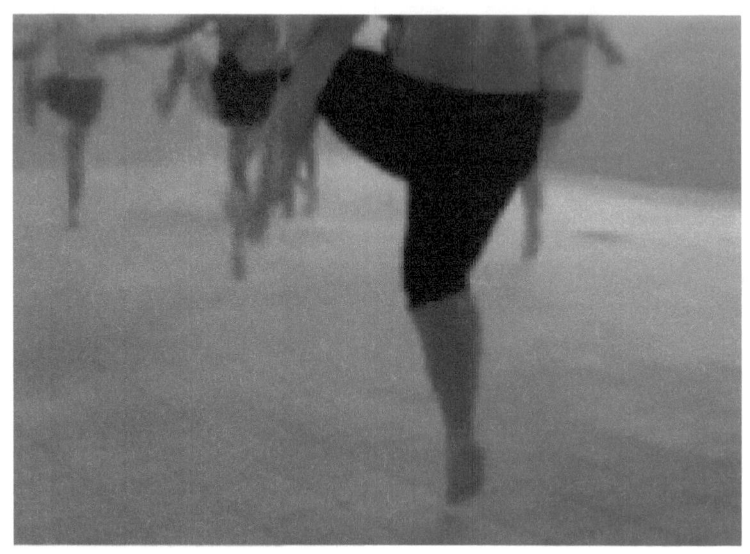

CALF RAISE

EQUIPMENT:

No equipment is needed.

BENEFIT:

This exercise helps to contract the calf muscles at the back of the lower leg.

PROCEDURE:

Firstly stand straight or upright. Ensure that your knees are straight. Raise your heel as high as possible. Return to the original position. 10-17 repetition. 2 sets.

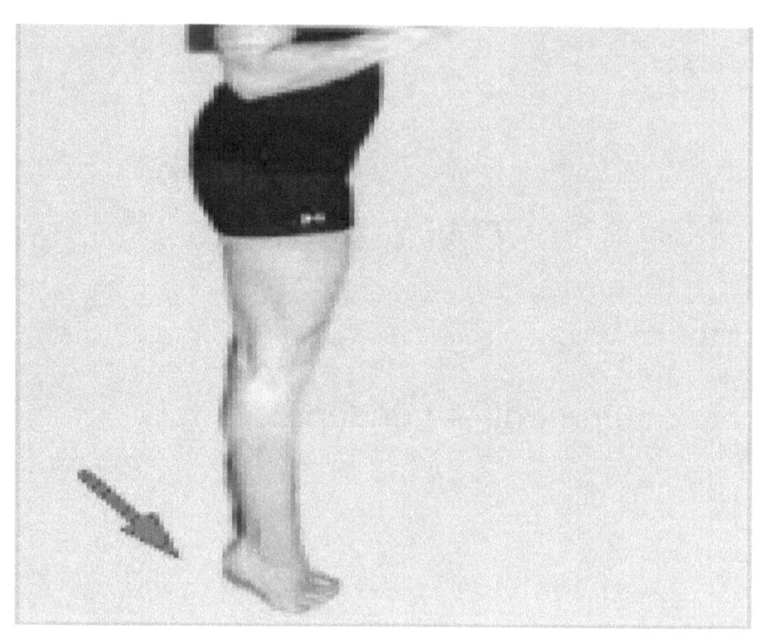

JUMPING JACK

EQUIPMENT:

No equipment is needed.

BENEFIT:

Improve your posture and strengthen muscles around your legs. It also boosts the inner as well as outer thigh and stabilizes your heart rate.

PROCEDURE:

This exercise is straightforward to do. Start by standing upright and your foot on the pool floor.

Jump upward direction with your feet above the floor while landing spread or widen your legs and return to the initial position by jumping upward again.

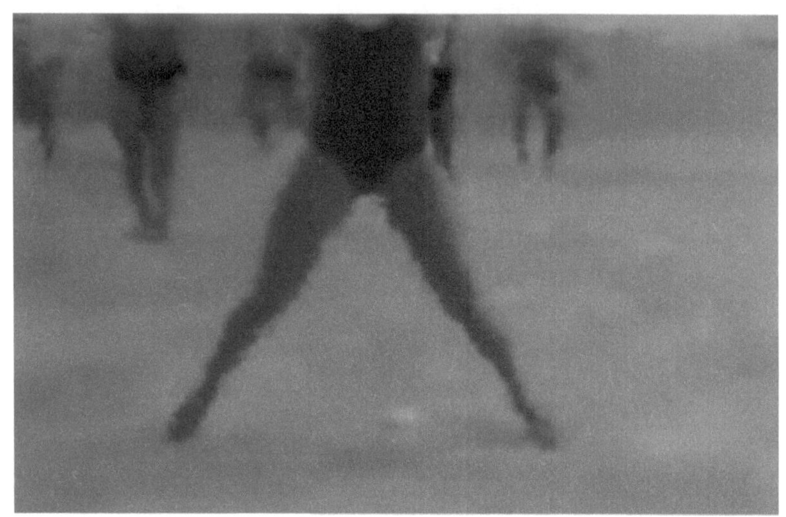

CROSS COUNTRY SKI

EQUIPMENT:

No equipment is needed.

BENEFIT:

It strengthens your shoulder muscles including the core part of your body and also improves your heart rate.

PROCEDURE:

Push off with both feet evenly as well as shift your leg posture in the air with a slight bounce using a knee bend. At the same time, land with both feet. To return to the initial position, repeat the procedure, this time changing your leg position.

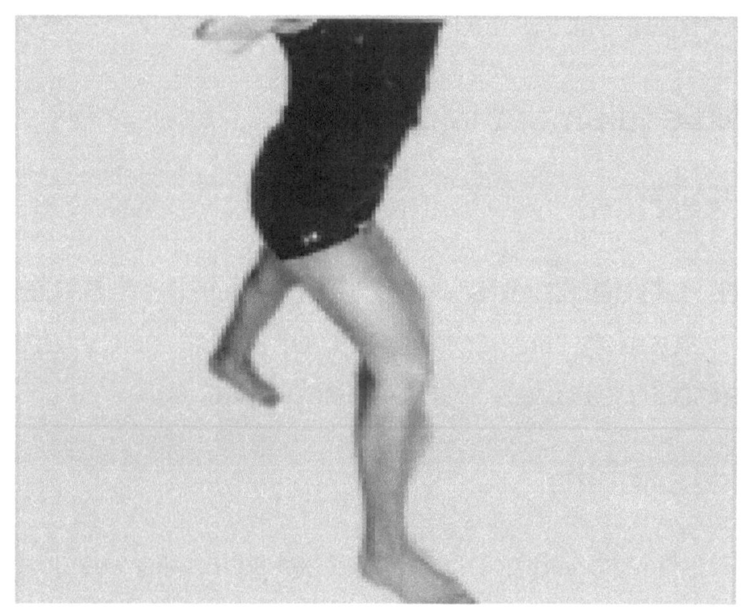

TRICEPS PUSH-DOWN

EQUIPMENT:

POOL NOODLE

BENEFIT:

It strengthens the triceps muscles at the back of the upper arm.

PROCEDURE:

- Start by standing upright in the pool and your foot on the floor of the pool.
- Hold on the pool noodle with your hands from the surface of the water.

- Then after pushing it down into the water and upward. Repeat 15-20 times.

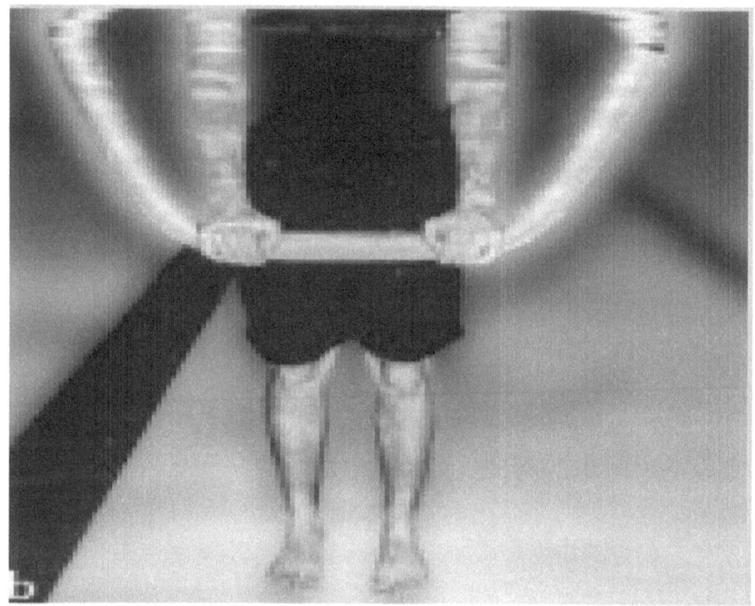

EXTERNAL SHOULDER ROTATION

EQUIPMENT:

No equipment is needed.

BENEFIT:

This exercise is best in strengthening the four muscles found in the shoulder rotator cuff.

PROCEDURE:

- Start by standing on the floor of the pool firmly.
- Your head and shoulder above the water surface.
- Bend your elbow 90 degrees and press strongly against the lower rib cage with fists in front of the body.

- Maintain both elbows pressed against the ribcage as well as extend the forearms away from the center of the torso as much as comfortably while keeping the elbows pressed against the ribcage. Return to the beginning.

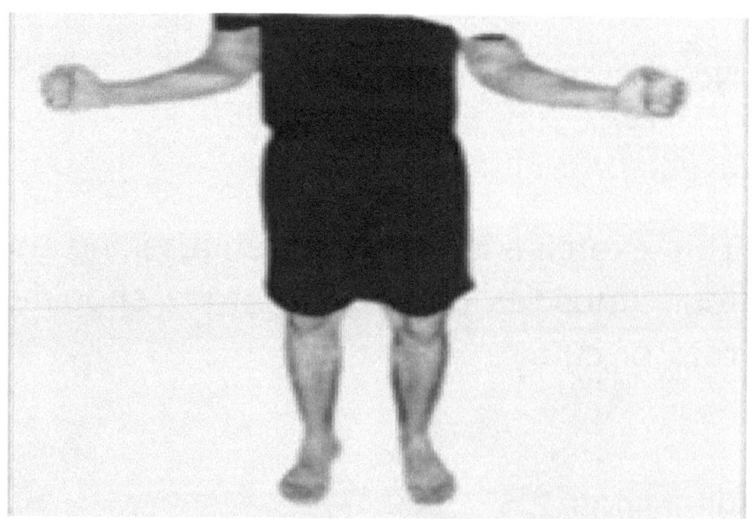

PUSH FRONT TO BACK

EQUIPMENT:

No equipment is needed.

BENEFIT:

Strengthen the knee joint, ankle, and hip. It strengthens the muscles in your leg.

PROCEDURE:

Firstly start by standing upright, your feet on the pool floor. Perform a jogging motion by raising your knee front and back by maintaining your fixed position.

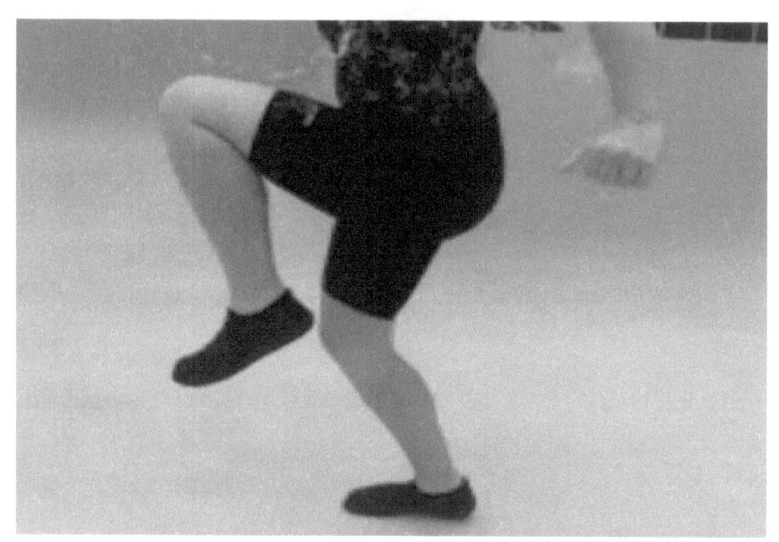

STRAIGHT LEG KICK TO THE FRONT

EQUIPMENT:

No equipment is needed.

BENEFIT:

It strengthens the muscles in the hip as well as the upper leg.

PROCEDURE:

- First, start by standing upright in the pool.
- Your legs should be on the pool floor.
- Raise your right leg 90 degrees.
- Your left leg bent a little as you tent to lower your body into the water.

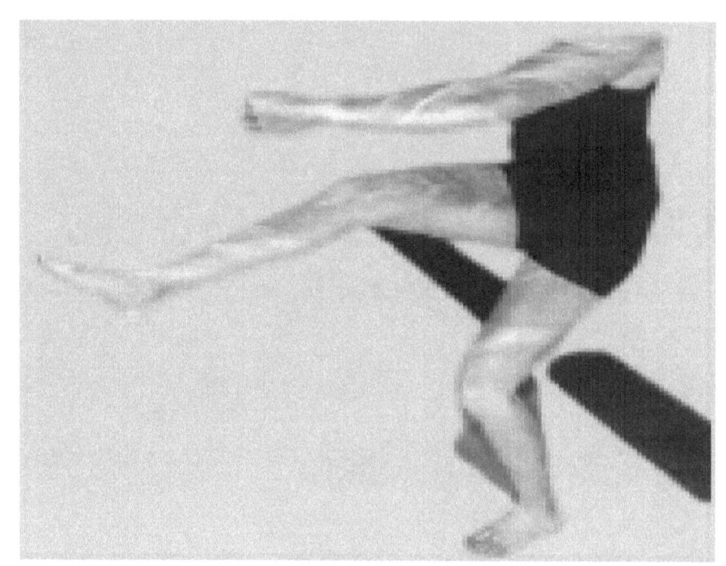

TRAVEL FORWARD

EQUIPMENT:

No equipment is needed.

BENEFIT:

It builds strong bones also strengthens the muscles.

PROCEDURE:

This is an easy exercise to do. It is just like land jogging but in this aspect, you are jogging right inside the pool by jogging in a forward direction.

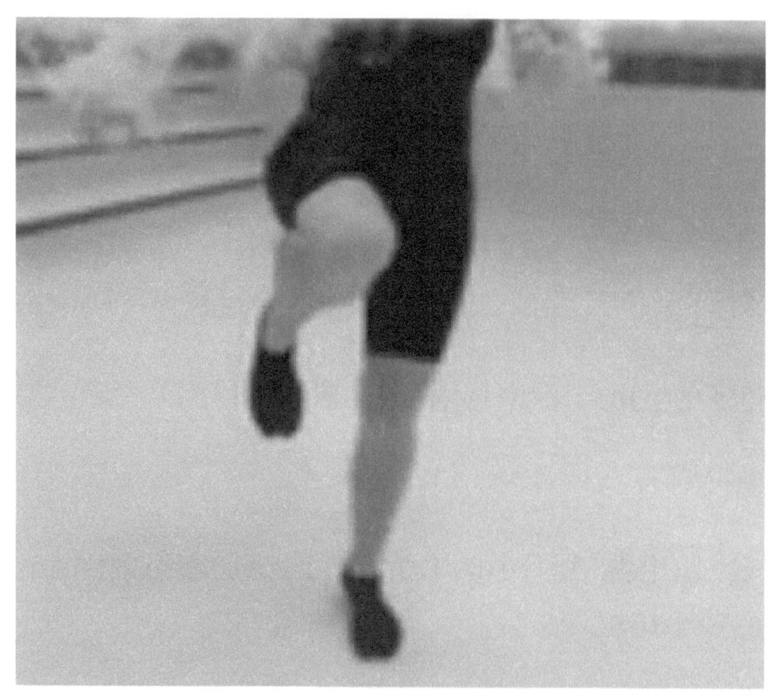

SIDE MOGUL

EQUIPMENT:

No equipment is needed.

BENEFIT:

Strengthen the muscles in the leg as well as as the core.

PROCEDURE:

Start by ensuring that your feet are jointly together, also make sure that you stand in the center of the pool with your head above the water and your foot on the pool floor and your hips forward, push off the pool floor as well as land with your feet jointly together and also slightly to the right side of your initial position.

Return to the starting position on the left side of the initial position by pushing off with both feet.

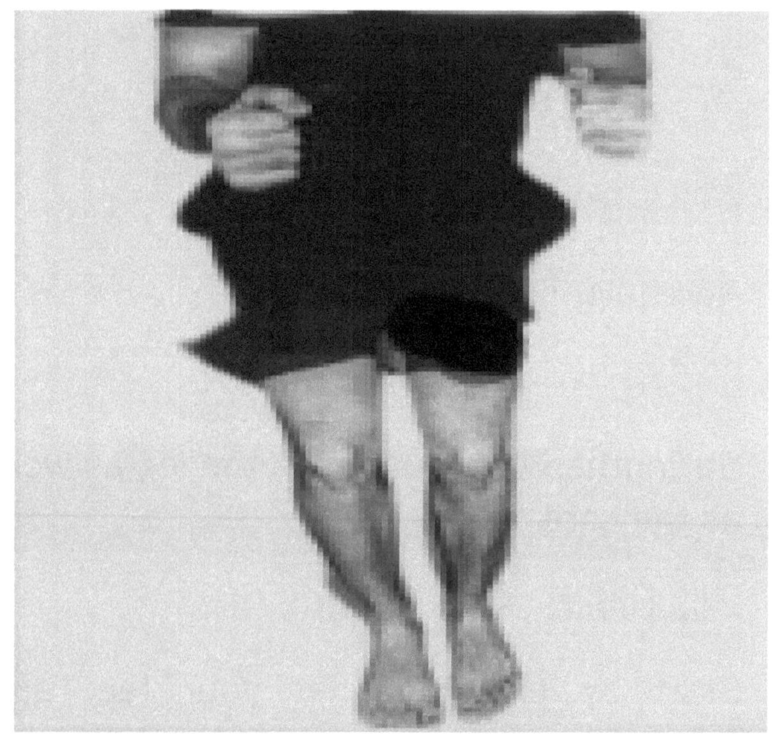

TWISTING MOGUL

EQUIPMENT:

No equipment is needed.

BENEFIT:

Strengthen the muscles in the leg as well as the core.

PROCEDURE:

First, stand upright in the center of the pool. Your feet on the floor of the pool and your head and shoulder above the water level.

Bend your knees, this will enable you to push off with your feet from the initial position after that rotate your body as well as land with both feet jointly together.

Push off both feet as well as rotate your body mostly to the left side, landing on both of your feet at a 45-degree angle to the left side.

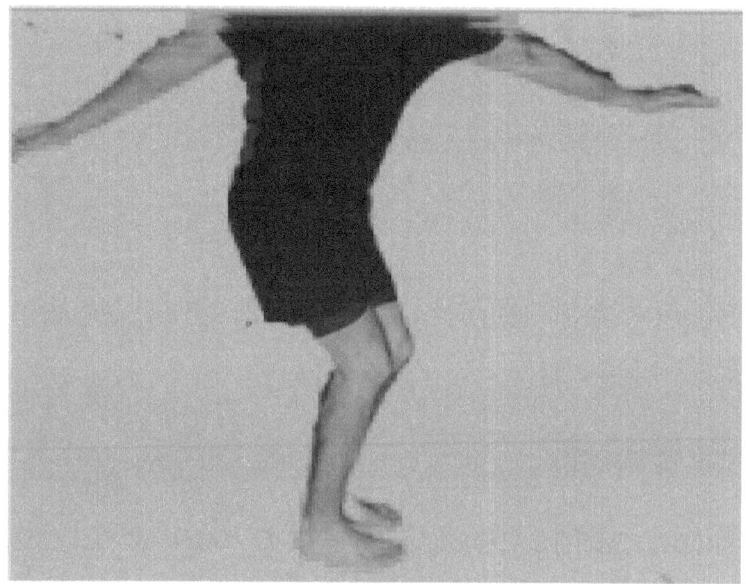

ARM SWING FRONT AND BACK

EQUIPMENT:

No equipment is needed.

BENEFIT:

Strengthen your muscles and your knee joint.

PROCEDURE:

Firstly start by standing upright, your feet on the pool floor. Perform a jogging motion by raising your knee front and back both legs by maintaining your fixed position then swing your hand front and backward direction as you continue to jog.

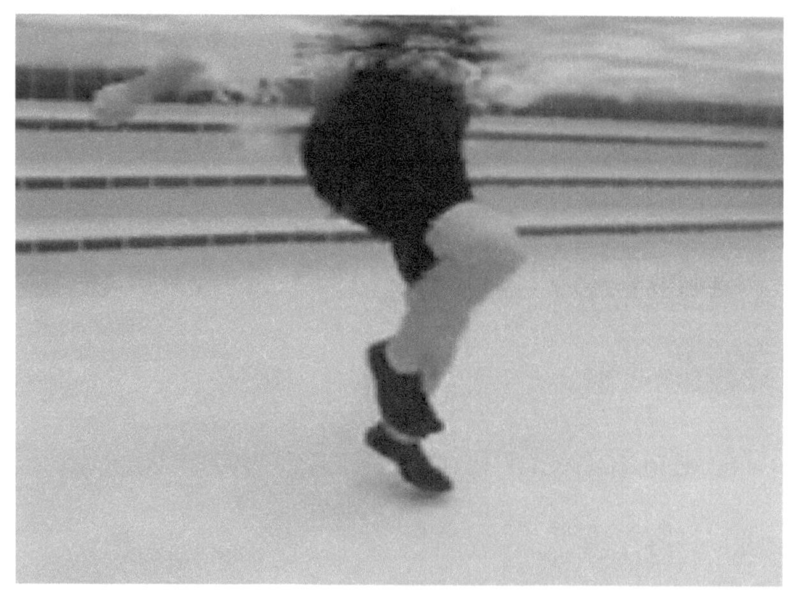